Everyday Wellness

Free Coaching Offer
Get a Free Coaching Call with the Author
of *Everyday Wellness*—See Page 121

Are You Making These Nine Common Health Mistakes?

Download Your Free Report
from www.lajollahealthcoach.com/ew

Everyday Wellness
Fifty Simple Steps to Lifelong Health

Marilyn Beidler

Foreword by Timothy Dooley, N.D., M.D.,
Author of *Homeopathy: Beyond Flat Earth Medicine*

La Jolla Health Coach

The purpose of this book is to educate, not to diagnose or treat any medical condition or to replace the counsel of a doctor or other qualified health professional. If you suspect that you have a medical problem, we urge you to seek competent medical help.

This book is sold with the understanding that the publisher and author shall have neither liability nor responsibility for any injury caused directly or indirectly by the information contained in this book. While every effort has been made to ensure the accuracy of this book, neither the author nor the publisher can be held responsible for errors or for the omission of pertinent information.

Copyright © 2009 by Marilyn Beidler.

All rights reserved. No part of this work may be reproduced, stored in a retrieval system, or transmitted in any form or by any means electronic, mechanical, photocopying, recording, or otherwise, without the prior permission of La Jolla Health Coach.

Printed in the United States of America

La Jolla Health Coach and the La Jolla Health Coach logo are trademarks of La Jolla Health Coach.

ISBN-13: 978-0-578-00569-0

For more information, or to order additional copies of this book, visit us on the web at www.lajollahealthcoach.com/everydaywellness

For my son, Joshua

Contents

Figures & Illustrations . . . . *iv*
Acknowledgements . . . . *v*
Foreword by Timothy Dooley, N.D., M.D. . . . . *vii*
Preface . . . . *ix*

SECTION 1: NOURISH 11
    1. Trim the Fat 13
    2. Downsize 15
    3. Play Good Carb, Bad Carb 17
    4. Put a Rainbow on Your Plate 19
    5. Break the Omega Code 21
    6. Join the Tribe 23
    7. Play It in Mono 25
    8. Snack Smarter 27
    9. Spice It Up 29
    10. Eat with the Seasons 31

i

Contents

SECTION 2: ENERGIZE 33
    1. Get S.M.A.R.T. 35
    2. Use the Buddy System 37
    3. Get Strong 39
    4. Flex Your Power 41
    5. Catch Your Z's 43
    6. Lighten Up 45
    7. Check Your Breaks 47
    8. Decaffeinate 49
    9. Listen to Your Heart 51
    10. Begin the Journey of 10,000 Steps 53

SECTION 3: PURIFY 55
    1. Filter It 57
    2. Don't Be a Softie 59
    3. A Better Bottle 61
    4. Just Breathe 63
    5. Filter It, Redux 65
    6. Spring Clean 67
    7. Catch That E.L.F. 69
    8. Take a Food Holiday 71
    9. Clean Up Your Act 73
    10. Discover Natural Beauty 75

Contents

SECTION 4: SIMPLIFY 77
   1. Simplify Your Schedule 79
   2. Singletask 81
   3. Go on a Media Diet 83
   4. Lower the Volume 85
   5. Unsubscribe 87
   6. Can the Clutter 89
   7. Give from the Heart 91
   8. Let Go 93
   9. Travel Light 95
   10. Celebrate Simply 97

SECTION 5: RENEW 99
   1. Go with the Flow 101
   2. Bring Nature Home 103
   3. Keep a Gratitude Journal 105
   4. Seek Solitude 107
   5. Cultivate Optimism 109
   6. Give Yourself a Time Out 111
   7. Destress Progressively 113
   8. Discover Your Signature Strengths 115
   9. Savor 117
   10. Renew Your Spirit 119

Figures & Illustrations

Figure 1. Foods High in Saturated Fat, and Healthier Alternatives. 12
Figure 2. Standard Serving Sizes 14
Figure 3. A Full Spectrum of Phytochemicals 18
Figure 4. Major Sources of Omega-3 and Omega-6 Fatty Acids 20
Figure 5. Major Sources of Monounsaturated Fats 24
Figure 6. Spices with Medicinal Properties 28
Figure 7. Activated Carbon and Reverse Osmosis Filters Compared 56
Figure 8. Soft Drinks by the Numbers 58
Figure 9. The Electromagnetic Spectrum 68
Figure 10. Commonly Allergic Foods 70

Key to Resources

◆ Book
◉ CD or DVD
▸ Web Site

Acknowledgements

Like any writing project, this book has been a collaborative effort. I wish to extend my gratitude to all those who made this work possible, including the authors and researchers upon whose hard work and occasional flashes of brilliance many of the suggestions in this book are based.

I would particularly like to thank Dr. Timothy Dooley, for writing an admirable foreword on rather short notice, and Dr. Brian Perks, for all his help over the years. Last but not least, I would like to thank my son, Joshua, who freely volunteered his support and encouragement during this demanding and time-consuming process.

As always, while many people deserve thanks for this book's successes, any errors it may contain are my responsibility alone.

Marilyn Beidler, C.N.C.

Foreword

An odd thing happened to me last month. I was riding my bicycle home (as I have done daily for years and years) and woke up in the hospital with an assortment of injuries and, in general, fairly banged up. I was in the hospital for three days, and during that time various friends and family members came to visit.

One of the angels who came to visit me was Marilyn Beidler, the author of this fine little book on wellness. The point is, Marilyn is one of those people who doesn't just talk, she does.

When she says people should walk 10,000 steps a day, she will show you her pedometer. When she says diet can improve your physical and mental health, she is speaking from years of experience and observation. And if you are lucky enough to hear her recommend planting a garden, get ready for piles of produce.

So don't wait until you are in the hospital with time on your hands to become acquainted with Marilyn through this book. Read it now—it will help you stay out of the hospital. That's my advice.

Timothy Dooley, N.D., M.D.,
Author of Homeopathy: Beyond Flat Earth Medicine
December 16, 2008

Preface

I chose the title *Everyday Wellness* deliberately. Although the words *health* and *wellness* are sometimes used interchangeably, wellness implies more than the absence of disease—it implies a positive state of optimal functioning.

In medicine, physicians still perform the necessary work of patching bones and curing infections. Today, however, many of us seek not only a longer lifespan, but also a longer "healthspan"—the length of time that one enjoys excellent health.

A second distinction is that wellness is holistic. It is concerned not only with the functioning of our physical bodies, but also with our thoughts, our relationships with others, and even our connection with the natural world.

The adjective *everyday* reminds us that achieving wellness is a lifelong effort. How we feel on our fortieth (or our eightieth) birthday is the result of thousands of decisions, few of which seem significant at the time.

The following pages describe fifty simple steps to greater health, fitness, serenity, and joy. This book is far from comprehensive: it would take a whole library of books to cover wellness thoroughly. But I believe that the most important thing isn't how far you've traveled in your journey, or how quickly, but that you're moving in the right direction. So whether your journey to wellness is well underway, or just beginning, I hope that this book will inspire you to keep placing one foot in front of the other.

Marilyn Beidler, C.N.C.
December 1, 2008

> "To eat is a necessity, but to eat intelligently is an art."
>
> La Rochefoucauld

Nourish

Fig. 1 Foods High in Saturated Fat, and Healthier Alternatives

INSTEAD OF THESE...	CHOOSE THESE INSTEAD...
Meats and Poultry	
Bacon	Chicken or turkey breast
Bologna	Beef, eye of round, lean only
Beef, 85% lean ground	Beef, 95% lean ground
Beef, sandwich steaks	Beef, top round, lean only
Salami	Turkey pastrami
Dairy and Eggs	
Most cheeses	Low-fat cottage cheese
Whole eggs	Egg whites
Whole or reduced-fat (2%) milk	Skim or low-fat (1%) milk
Nuts and Seeds	
Brazil nuts	Almonds
Coconut	Walnuts
Fats and Oils	
Butter	Almond oil
Coconut oil	Avocado oil
Cottonseed oil	Canola oil
Palm or palm kernel oil	High-oleic safflower or sunflower oil
Peanut oil	Olive oil

1 TRIM THE FAT.

I know, you've heard it before. But the U.S. government and many health organizations agree that limiting fat to 30 percent of our caloric intake is one of the most important things we can do for our health. That's because a high-fat diet is an important risk factor for cardiovascular disease, diabetes, obesity, and cancers of the breast, colon, and prostate.

Not all fats are equally bad, however. The worst culprit is trans fat, which greatly increases your risk of developing coronary heart disease, and may also promote Alzheimer's disease, cancer, and diabetes. In the United States, a food can legally be advertised as free of trans fat if it contains less than half a gram of trans fat per serving. Unfortunately, many small servings can add up to a substantial amount of trans fat per day. To minimize trans fat consumption, check the ingredients list and don't eat anything that contains *hydrogenated vegetable oil, partially hydrogenated vegetable oil,* or *shortening.* When you dine out, ask your server if the food contains any of these ingredients.

The other fat to avoid is saturated fat, which raises blood cholesterol and increases your risk of developing atherosclerosis and coronary heart disease. You can reduce your saturated fat intake by choosing monounsaturated oils and reducing your consumption of meat and dairy. When you do eat meat or dairy products, choose lean, low-fat, and non-fat versions.

LEARN MORE

◆ *The Omega Diet,* Artemis P. Simopoulos and Jo Robinson
▸ *Nutrient Search Tool* (www.nutritiondata.com/tools/nutrient-search)

Fig. 2   Standard Serving Sizes

Meat, Poultry, and Fish

2 to 3 ounces of meat (about the size of a deck of playing cards)

1 chicken breast

1 medium pork chop

¼ lb hamburger patty

2½ to 3 ounces of edible fish or seafood (equivalent to ¾ lb whole fish or ½ lb dressed fish or fish with bones)

Dairy Products

1 cup yogurt or milk

1½ ounces of cheddar cheese

Grains and Legumes

1 slice of whole-grain bread

½ cup of cooked rice or pasta

½ cup of mashed potatoes

3 to 4 small crackers

1 small pancake or waffle

2 medium-sized cookies

Fruits and Vegetables

½ cup cooked vegetables

1 cup (4 leaves) lettuce

1 small baked potato

¾ cup vegetable juice

1 medium apple

½ grapefruit or mango

½ cup berries

2 Downsize.

Remember legwarmers, synthesizer pop, and the side ponytail? The Me Decade left us with another legacy most of us wish we could forget—that was when portion sizes ballooned out of control, and so did our waistlines.

Since the 1950s, the number of calories in the largest-size bottle of Coca-Cola has more than doubled. The caloric content of the largest Snickers bar has more than tripled. Convenience stores serve soft drinks in 64-ounce cups. And even most table-service restaurants have switched from ten-inch to twelve-inch plates.

Supersized portions wouldn't be a problem if we only ate when we were hungry and stopped eating when we're full. Unfortunately, studies have shown that we consume up to 30 percent more calories when we're served larger portions. Not surprisingly, our total caloric intake has gone up. The average American man consumes 168 more calories per day than his counterpart did in 1970; the average American woman consumes 335 more calories.

To get a handle on your caloric intake, pay close attention to suggested serving sizes. That bag of chips you just ate in one sitting may have been labeled for a dozen servings. When you dine out, order an appetizer or half-portion, split an entrée with a companion, or take half of it home with you. When you eat at home, take a reasonable portion, then wait twenty minutes. You may be surprised how often you won't need to go back for seconds.

Learn More

- *The Fattening of America*, Eric A. Finkelstein
- *Mindless Eating*, Brian Wansink

Nourish

"Sugar is a type of bodily fuel, yes, but your body runs about as well on it as a car would."

V. L. ALLINEARE

3 Play Good Carb, Bad Carb.

If you're confused about carbohydrates, you have plenty of company. In the eighties we thought fat was public enemy number one, so we loaded up on breads, pasta, and fat-free snacks. (Who could resist the prospect of enjoying chocolate cupcakes with a clear conscience? The only problem was that they usually tasted like sawdust.)

Then came the nineties, and the low-carb craze got underway. Fat was given a suspended sentence, while carbs took the rap for our high cholesterol and expanding waistlines.

As usual, the truth is more complex than the diet books let on. Protein, fat, and carbohydrates are all essential components of a healthy diet. And just as some fats increase our risk of chronic disease, while others lower it, the same holds true of carbohydrates.

In the "bad carb" category are refined grains, like white flour and white rice, and sweeteners, like sugar and high-fructose corn syrup. Virtually devoid of vitamins and minerals, these foods are also low in fiber, so it's easy to take in a lot of calories without feeling satisfied. Not surprisingly, they put us at greater risk of obesity, insulin resistance, diabetes, and cardiovascular disease.

In the "good carb" category are whole grains and legumes, fruits and vegetables. These high-fiber foods can actually lower cholesterol and reduce your risk of certain cancers. It's important to keep in mind, however, that too much of a good thing is still too much. Eat even whole grains in moderation, especially if you're trying to lose weight or lower your triglycerides.

Learn More

▸ *Whole Grains Fact Sheet*
(www.ific.org/publications/factsheets/wholegrainsfs.cfm)

Fig. 3 A Full Spectrum of Phytochemicals

To Get More...	Think...
Anthocyanidins May protect collagen.	*Blue:* Blueberries *Red:* Cherries, raspberries *Black:* Blackberries
Carotenes Important for eye health.	*Dark green:* Beet greens, collard greens, kale, spinach *Yellow:* Peppers, sweet potatoes *Orange:* Apricots, butternut squash, cantaloupe, carrots, mangos, pumpkins, yams
Ellagic acid May help prevent cancer.	*Red:* Apples, raspberries, strawberries *Purple:* Grapes
Limonoids May help prevent cancer.	*Yellow:* Lemons, other citrus fruits
Lutein May promote eye health.	*Dark green:* Collard greens, kale, spinach, swiss chard
Lycopene May promote prostate health.	*Red:* Guava, pink grapefruit, red peppers, tomatoes, watermelon
Resveratrol May lower blood sugar and help prevent cancer.	*Red:* Grapes, mulberries, red wine
Quercetin May help prevent cancer.	*Red:* Apples, cherries, cranberries, peppers *White:* Onions

4 Put a Rainbow on Your Plate.

Fruits and vegetables are the heart of a healthy diet. Unfortunately, fewer than a quarter of Americans follow the government's recommendation to eat five servings of fruits and vegetables per day. If you're part of that virtuous minority, don't turn the page just yet; five servings a day is a good start, but it's still not enough for optimal nutrition.

Research has shown that a diet rich in fruits and vegetables is associated with a lower risk of many chronic diseases, including coronary heart disease, stroke, type II diabetes, and certain cancers. Fruits and vegetables are the unsung heroes of nutrition—low in calories and fat, but packed with vitamins, minerals, and hundreds of beneficial phytochemicals.

Salads are a convenient way to get more vegetables into your diet. But don't stop with lettuce—try adding finely chopped beet greens, kale, or swiss chard, sliced tomatoes or red bell peppers, green onions, and grated carrots or beets. Add a little salad dressing, or make your own from a tablespoon of olive oil, the juice from half a lemon, a pinch of stevia, and your favorite herbs.

Because different nutrients pick different fruits and vegetables to hang out in, you'll have a better chance of getting a full spectrum of nutrients if you eat a whole rainbow of colors. (Yes, white is a color. And no, frosting doesn't count.)

Learn More

◆ *Vegetables from Amaranth to Zucchini*, Elizabeth Schneider
◆ *Vegetables Every Day*, Jack Bishop

Fig. 4 Major Sources of Omega-3 and Omega-6 Fatty Acids

INCREASE INTAKE OF FOODS HIGH IN OMEGA-3

Fish and Seafood

Anchovies	Mackerel	Shark
Bluefish	Sablefish	Trout
Dogfish	Salmon	Tuna (packed in water)
Herring	Sardines (packed in water)	Whitefish
Lake trout	Shad	

Nuts and Seeds

Chia seeds	Flax seeds	Walnuts

Fats and Oils

Canola oil	Flaxseed oil	Walnut oil

REDUCE INTAKE OF FOODS HIGH IN OMEGA-6

Nuts and Seeds

Brazil nuts	Pine nuts (pignolias)	Sesame seeds
Pecans	Pumpkin seeds (pepitas)	Sunflower seeds

Fats and Oils

Corn oil	Margarine	Rice bran oil
Cottonseed oil	Peanut oil	Sesame oil
Grapeseed oil	Poppyseed oil	Soybean oil

5 Break the Omega Code.

Remember when replacing saturated fat with polyunsaturated vegetable oils was the health-conscious thing to do? The truth turns out to be slightly more complicated. Polyunsaturated fats come in omega-3 and omega-6 versions. And while our Paleolithic ancestors consumed the two types of fat in nearly equal proportions, most Americans get fourteen to twenty times more omega-6 than omega-3. This high omega-6 to omega-3 ratio has been linked to increased risk for many serious diseases, including heart disease, stroke, cancer, diabetes, arthritis, depression, and Alzheimer's disease.

What can you do to improve your fat IQ? Start by eating two or more 2½- to 3-ounce servings of fatty fish per week. (Lean fish and seafood are great sources of protein, but not of omega-3 fatty acids.) If you buy canned tuna, make sure it's not a reduced-fat variety, and that it's packed in water instead of oil. Vegetarian options include chia seeds sprinkled on your breakfast cereal, flaxseed meal in baked goods, and walnuts as a snack. Flaxseed oil is unsuitable for cooking, but fine for salad dressings.

EPA and DHA are two particularly important omega-3 fatty acids found in fish. If you don't like fish, consider taking a fish oil supplement that provides a total daily dose of 1,000 mg EPA and DHA. Plant-based sources of EPA and DHA are few and far between, but some companies are now selling algae-based supplements that are 100 percent vegan.

LEARN MORE

◆ *The Omega-3 Connection*, Andrew Stoll
◆ *The Omega Diet*, Artemis P. Simopoulos, M.D., and Jo Robinson

"Human consciousness arose but a minute before midnight on the geological clock. Yet we mayflies try to bend an ancient world to our purposes, ignorant perhaps of the messages buried in its long history."

STEPHEN JAY GOULD

6 JOIN THE TRIBE.

If all of human existence were compressed into a single day, we would have been hunter-gatherers for the first 23 hours and 52 minutes. Agriculture would have existed for a little over seven minutes, and the industrial age for less than nine seconds. But while the way we live our lives has changed dramatically within just the past decade, we share 99.99 percent of our genes with Cro-Magnon mammoth-hunters who roamed Europe some 40,000 years ago.

Proponents of the Paleolithic diet believe that many of our modern health problems are the result of a mismatch between our ancient genes and our modern environment. Early humans didn't eat grains or dairy products, but they had strong bones because they consumed plenty of calcium-rich vegetables. Other dietary staples included fruits, lean meats, fish, and nuts and seeds. Water was their only beverage, and honey their only sweetener, which they enjoyed occasionally at the price of painful stings.

Fresh air, daily physical activity, and plentiful social support rounded out a lifestyle that modern humans would do well to learn from. And while it would be difficult for us to adopt the Paleolithic lifestyle in its entirety, we can at least eat more whole foods and ditch our cell phones once in a while.

LEARN MORE

◆ *The Paleo Diet,* Loren Cordain
◆ *The Paleolithic Prescription,* S. Boyd Eaton, Marjorie Shostak, and Melvin Konner

Fig. 5 Major Sources of Monounsaturated Fat

Fruits and Vegetables

Avocados	Olives

Nuts and Seeds

Almonds	Peanut butter
Cashews	Peanuts
Hazelnuts (filberts)	Pecans
Hickory nuts	Pistachio nuts
Macadamia nuts	

Fats and Oils

Almond oil	High-oleic safflower oil
Avocado oil	High-oleic sunflower oil
Canola oil	Olive oil
Hazelnut oil	

7 Play It in Mono.

Move over, polyunsaturated vegetable oils. Placing a greater emphasis on monounsaturated oils could be one of the most important things you'll ever do for your heart.

In the 1960s, the influential Keys study discovered that the men of Crete had half the cancer rate and just one twentieth the mortality from coronary artery disease as their American counterparts. Many researchers believe that olive oil, a rich source of monounsaturated fat, is a major reason for the health benefits of the Mediterranean diet. Monounsaturated oils are the only type of fat proven to lower blood levels of harmful LDL cholesterol while maintaining or even raising levels of beneficial HDL cholesterol.

So toss out that bottle of corn or soybean oil and start cooking with monounsaturated oils instead. Use olive oil to impart a distinctive flavor to stews, sautés, and salad dressings. In desserts and other foods that call for a more delicate touch, use canola oil. Safflower oil and sunflower oil are also acceptable, but only if they're labeled *high-oleic*—the conventional versions of these oils contain mostly omega-6 polyunsaturated fats, which may increase one's risk of cancer and cardiovascular disease when consumed in the large quantities typically found in the American diet.

At the store, look for packaged foods made with canola oil. And when you eat out, don't forget to ask what kind of oil they use in the kitchen. More and more restaurants are making the switch to heart-healthy monounsaturated oils.

Learn More

◆ *Fats and Oils,* Udo Erasmus
◆ *The Omega Diet,* Artemis P. Simopoulos, M.D., and Jo Robinson

*"If junk food is the devil,
then a sweet orange
is as scripture."*

AUDREY FORIS

8 SNACK SMARTER.

These days, few of us feel we have time to sit down for three leisurely meals. Snacking is a better fit for our busy schedules. Unfortunately, it may not be a good fit for our biology.

For most of our evolutionary history, we humans followed most of our meals with several hours of fasting. When we snack too often (or sip soft drinks between meals), we ensure that our blood sugar levels stay elevated. High blood sugar leads to increased production of insulin, which triggers our bodies to store food energy as fat. We may also be more likely to develop insulin resistance, a condition that often progresses to diabetes.

What can you do to keep your blood sugar levels on a natural cycle? Start by eating three solid meals every day. Snack only if you're hungry, not just because you're bored. (This rule also applies to milk, soft drinks and all other beverages that contain fat or sugar.)

When you really are hungry between meals, go ahead and have a healthy snack. Enjoy fresh fruit, or blenderize frozen fruit with skim milk for a frosty treat. Slice raw vegetables and dip them in hummus or nut butter. Have a slice of whole-grain bread with a piece of skinless chicken breast. Or add some fresh fruit to a single-serving container of plain low-fat yogurt. With a little creativity, snacks can be healthy as well as convenient.

LEARN MORE

▸ *The Healthy Snacks Blog* (www.thehealthysnacksblog.com)

Fig. 6 Spices with Medicinal Properties

Herb or Spice	Cuisines	Traditional Uses
Allspice	Caribbean, Middle Eastern	Colds, fatigue, gas, sinus congestion
Anise seed	European	Colds, coughs, gas, indigestion, insomnia, menstrual cramps
Basil	Chinese, Italian	Anxiety, headaches, indigestion
Black pepper	European, Indian	Boils, cough, indigestion
Cardamom	Indian, Middle Eastern, Nordic	Congestion, colds, coughs, diarrhea, indigestion, nausea
Cinnamon	European, Middle Eastern	Colds, indigestion, toothache
Coriander seed	Indian	Indigestion, rheumatism
Cumin	Indian, Middle Eastern	Aphrodisiac, coughs, gas, indigestion
Fennel	Indian, Italian, Middle Eastern	Suppressing appetite, indigestion, menopausal symptoms
Fenugreek	Indian, Middle Eastern	Congestion, increasing lactation, ulcers and stomach problems
Peppermint	English, Middle Eastern	Indigestion, menstrual cramps
Rosemary	English, Mediterranean	Colds, indigestion, headache
Tarragon	French	Anxiety, indigestion, insomnia
Turmeric	Indian, Middle Eastern	Indigestion, liver health

9 Spice It Up.

Herbs and spices are the double agents of the food world. You may know them as versatile seasonings that make food fun without running up your daily totals of calories, fat, and sodium. But many of these same herbs and spices occupy a central place in traditional Chinese and Ayurvedic medicine. Here are four of the most promising:

- *Cinnamon.* Native to Sri Lanka, cinnamon was being imported to Egypt as early as 2,000 B.C.E. It is one of the fifty essential herbs in Chinese medicine, and as little as ½ teaspoon has been found to lower blood sugar levels.
- *Garlic.* Used as a medicine for thousands of years, garlic has been investigated for possible cardiovascular benefits. It may also help regulate blood sugar levels and fight infection. Garlic's benefits may be enhanced by cooking it with tomato.
- *Ginger.* In Chinese herbal medicine, ginger is used to support the stomach, spleen, heart, lungs, and kidneys. Westerners have used ginger as a digestive aid, and to treat nausea caused by seasickness, morning sickness, or chemotherapy.
- *Turmeric.* A staple of Indian cooking, turmeric is also used as an antiseptic. Turmeric's active ingredient, curcumin, may help prevent Alzheimer's disease and diabetes, fight cancer, and soothe inflammation in people with arthritis.

Learn More

◆ *Encyclopedia of Medicinal Plants*, Andrew Chevallier
◆ *The Healing Cuisine: India's Art of Ayurvedic Cooking*, Harish Johari

*"In seed time learn,
in harvest teach,
in winter enjoy."*

WILLIAM BLAKE

10 Eat with the Seasons.

Most of us never think about the global network of jet planes, cargo ships, and big-rig trucks that keeps the local supermarket stocked with exotic delicacies. On a typical day, you might find grapes from Chile, cilantro from Costa Rica, cantaloupes from Ecuador, and kiwi fruits from South Africa.

As marvelous as this bounty is, however, more and more people are raising questions about the drawbacks of our globalized food supply. For one thing, shipping food halfway around the world uses a lot of fuel. In fact, importing food can generate 650 times as much carbon dioxide as growing it locally! Safety is another concern, since food is often imported from countries whose standards are not as strict as those in the United States.

In contrast, eating locally supports the local economy and reduces our impact on the environment. It also increases our awareness of the earth and of the passage of time, as each season graces our kitchen tables with a different harvest.

Spring, the season of growth and renewal, brings an abundance of fresh greens that gently cleanse our bodies. The bounty of fresh fruits and vegetables reaches its peak during the balmy summer months, when salads and fresh fruit help us cool down. The autumn harvest brings nuts, squash, and root vegetables, which provide hearty nourishment through the cold winter months.

To eat in closer harmony with the seasons, shop regularly for fresh produce at your grocery store or farmer's market. Bring a grocery list, but be flexible. Look for recipes that incorporate seasonal ingredients, and adapt your favorite dishes to include whatever foods are in season at the moment.

Learn More

- *A Cookbook for All Seasons*, Elson M. Haas and Eleaonora Manzolini
- *Staying Healthy with the Seasons*, Elson M. Haas
- *FoodRoutes* (www.foodroutes.org)

> "*Energy creates energy.
> It is by spending oneself
> that one becomes rich.*"
>
> — Sarah Bernhardt

Energize

"A goal without a plan is just a wish."

Antoine de Saint-Exupery

1 Get S.M.A.R.T.

If you have trouble sticking with your workout program, you might want to take a good look at your goals. Are they clear? Are they realistic? Do they inspire you to be your best? Whether you want to lose weight, gain muscle, or compete in a triathlon, planning can greatly increase your chances of success.

In the business world, consultants often use the acronym S.M.A.R.T. to help companies design better goals. You can use the same concept to improve your health and fitness. There are many variations on the S.M.A.R.T. formula, but the five letters are usually taken to mean *Specific, Measurable, Attainable, Realistic* and *Timely*. Let's take a closer look at each of these terms:

- *Specific* means that a goal is clearly defined, not subject to interpretation. A vague goal such as "getting in shape" is less powerful than a specific goal such as "reducing my waist measurement by two inches."
- *Measurable* means that you track your progress using numbers, such as miles walked or calories consumed. Remember, you can't manage what you don't measure.
- *Attainable* and *Realistic* mean that the goal is something you can achieve. In other words, if you were a couch potato until this morning, don't try to run a marathon three months from now.
- *Timely* means that you have set a deadline by which you expect to accomplish your goal. Setting a date creates a sense of urgency and gives you something to strive for.

Learn More

◆ *Breaking the Pattern*, Charles Stuart Platkin

"My best friend is the one who brings out the best in me."

Henry Ford

2 Use the Buddy System.

Forget cyclometers and fancy running shoes—an exercise partner could be your most useful fitness accessory. Having a workout buddy makes exercise more fun by letting you socialize while you sweat. And having someone to hold you accountable can help motivate you to keep showing up, even on those cold mornings when it would be easier to stay in bed. (A little healthy competition can also boost your motivation.)

Don't have an exercise buddy, and don't know where to look? You could do worse than to recruit a friend or family member—just make sure that he or she is interested in working out as well as chatting.

If none of your friends are willing to get off the couch, try joining a fitness group or posting a note on the message board at your nearest gym, medical center, or sports equipment store. And if all else fails, several websites can introduce you to fellow fitness enthusiasts.

Remember to be specific about what you're looking for, and make sure your interests and level of fitness are compatible. (If you're just starting a walking program, don't work out with a seasoned triathlete, or vice versa.) If you're a woman, you can avoid unwanted attention by specifying that you're not looking for a date. And as always, use common sense when meeting strangers for the first time.

Learn More

- *ExerciseFriends.com* (www.exercisefriends.com)
- *Meetup.com* (www.meetup.com)
- *ReadyToSweat.com* (www.readytosweat.com)

*"The undertaking
of a new action brings
new strength."*

Evenius

3 GET STRONG.

If you're like most people, the term "strength training" conjures up a mental image of young male bodybuilders bench-pressing hundreds of pounds while hard rock blares through gym speakers. Stereotypes aside, strength training has important benefits for adults of both genders and all ages.

If you're a woman, strength training will help you stave off osteoporosis by increasing your bone density. Afraid you'll bulk up? Don't be. Unless you lift weights all day long, you'll never look like Arnold Schwarzenegger. But strength training *will* improve your muscle tone, giving you a sleeker and more youthful appearance.

If you're an older adult, strength training can reduce your risk of muscle injury, helping you to avoid disability and live independently longer.

And while aerobic exercise is more effective at burning calories, strength training can be a useful adjunct for those trying to lose weight. Dieters often lose more muscle than fat, but adding a strength training component to your exercise program will help you maintain muscle mass.

Don't have a gym membership or an expensive weight machine? Then work out at home with inexpensive dumbbells, kettlebells, clubbells, medicine balls, or resistance bands. Once you have your doctor's okay, you can train two or three days a week. Perform one set of each exercise, with eight to ten repetitions per set. (For beginners, one set provides nearly as much benefit as multiple sets.) When you can perform more than ten repetitions, you're ready to move up to a slightly heavier weight.

LEARN MORE

◆ *The New Rules of Lifting for Women*, Lou Schuler and Cassandra Forsythe
◆ *Strength Training Over 50*, D. Cristine Caivano

"Yoga is the fountain of youth. You're only as young as your spine is flexible."

Bob Harper

4 Flex Your Power.

When you design your exercise program, it's easy to focus on endurance or strength training and forget about the benefits of flexibility. That's too bad, because exercising for flexibility can improve your posture, lubricate your joints, reduce your risk of injury, and help you maintain a full range of motion as you grow older.

Pilates, tai chi, and yoga are all good ways to increase flexibility. Aim for three sessions a week, and remember to slow down and take your time; a few hasty stretches are unlikely to do much good, and could lead to injury.

It's also important to warm up before exercising and to cool down afterwards. The best way to warm up is simply to perform your usual exercise at a slower pace. Your warm-up time should vary depending on the ambient temperature. On warm days, five minutes may be enough. On cold days, you may need fifteen. To cool down, follow three to five minutes of walking with stretching or other flexibility exercises.

Learn More

- *Light on Yoga*, B. K. S. Iyengar and Yehudi Menuhin
- *Sunrise Tai Chi*, Ramel Rones (DVD)
- *Yoga For Beginners*, Barbara Benagh (DVD)

*"Work eight hours
and sleep eight hours
and make sure that they
are not the same hours."*

T. Boone Pickens

5 Catch Your Z's.

Americans get about six and a half hours of sleep each night, about an hour less than we averaged in the 1950s. Blame long hours at work, nearly an hour a day spent commuting, and a proliferation of late-night television shows that tempt us to stay up late. But our poor sleeping habits come at a price. Not getting adequate sleep greatly increases our risk of deadly accidents, and may even cause us to gain weight more easily.

Millions of Americans suffer from sleep-related conditions, such as sleep apnea, that require medical treatment. The rest of us can improve the quality of our sleep by taking a few simple steps on our own:

- *Try to go to bed and wake up at the same time every day*—even on weekends.
- *Avoid drinking coffee, tea, or caffeinated soft drinks after lunch.*
- *Make sure your bedroom is dark and quiet.* If you need to, buy blackout shades and a white noise machine.
- *Do something relaxing for an hour before bed,* like reading a novel or listening to soothing music, but avoid stimulating activities such as working, studying, or watching TV.
- *Avoid exercising right before bed.* On the other hand, exercising vigorously earlier in the evening can actually promote sleep by increasing the temperature of your brain, which creates a compensatory drop in temperature about four hours later. A hot bath four hours before you go to bed often has the same effect.

Learn More

◆ *The Insomnia Answer,* Paul Glovinsky and Art Spielman
➤ *National Sleep Foundation* (www.sleepfoundation.org)

Energize **43**

"There is a muscular energy in sunlight corresponding to the spiritual energy of wind."

Annie Dillard

6 Lighten Up.

If there's one thing we can count on, it's the sun. Rising and setting as reliably as clockwork, it's easy to take for granted. Yet none of us would be here without it, and growing evidence underscores just how important sunlight is for our health.

Sunlight triggers the production of vitamin D, a hormone which plays a crucial role in our health by promoting bone density and preventing cancer. When we spend most of our time indoors and wear sunscreen when we go out, we may not produce enough vitamin D for optimal health. Ultraviolet-B, the wavelength that triggers vitamin D production, is blocked by clothing, sunscreen, and glass.

A second benefit of natural light is that it promotes normal mood and a healthy sleep cycle by resetting our internal clocks. (Indoor lighting may not be sufficiently intense to perform this function.)

Our ancestors got plenty of sunlight because they spent much of their lives outdoors. In contrast, many modern humans rarely leave the shelter of our homes, offices, and indoor malls. In recent years, legitimate concerns about skin cancer have led some people to shun sunlight altogether.

Fortunately, it's possible to avoid sunburn while still getting the benefits of natural light. Begin each day by exposing your eyes and skin to sunlight for ten minutes. Never look directly at the sun, go inside before your skin becomes pink, and limit sun exposure between 10:00 A.M. and 2:00 P.M., when the sun's rays are at their most intense.

Learn More

◆ *Light: Medicine of the Future,* Jacob Liberman
◆ *The UV Advantage,* Michael Holick

*"Sometimes the most urgent
thing you can possibly do
is take a complete rest."*

Ashleigh Brilliant

7 Check Your Breaks.

It may sound paradoxical, but you'll get more done if you periodically take a break from your work. Getting up from your desk and stretching your limbs for a few minutes can improve your posture, relieve eye strain, and help you return to the task at hand with renewed focus and enthusiasm. Here are a few ideas to help you recharge your batteries:

- *Take a walk during your lunch break.* Even fifteen or twenty minutes will boost your daily step count and help you get some distance from the stresses of work. Your walking break will be even more effective if you can spend a few minutes in a nearby park or tree-lined courtyard; studies have shown that time spent in nature is a powerful way to increase positive emotions and improve concentration.
- *Beat the afternoon slump.* If you usually reach for coffee and doughnuts around 2:00 P.M., try a healthy snack followed by a quick nap or meditation exercise. Or get up and dance or do some jumping jacks. (This last suggestion is easier to put into practice if you work from a home office.)
- *Let your computer be your coach.* If you spend a lot of time working on a computer, you can download a free program that will remind you to take breaks. In addition to increasing your energy level, you'll also reduce your risk of Repetitive Stress Injuries.

Learn More

- *AntiRSI* (Mac OS X) (tech.inhelsinki.nl/antirsi)
- *Workrave* (Linux, Windows) (www.workrave.org)

"Widespread caffeine use explains a lot about the twentieth century."

Greg Egan

8 DECAFFEINATE.

These days, it seems that most of us are trying to do more in less time. When we're under more pressure than the contents of an espresso maker, it's second nature to reach for a caffeinated pick-me-up. In recent years, the old-fashioned cup of joe (caffeine content: about 100 mg) has been joined by an assortment of coffee drinks, soft drinks, and energy drinks, some of which pack a whopping 500 mg of caffeine.

While an occasional dose of caffeine is probably harmless, too much can lead to serious health problems. In addition to being mildly addictive, caffeine is capable of causing nervousness, irritability, insomnia, headaches, and heart palpitations. It also promotes calcium loss, potentially increasing your risk of osteoporosis. And although caffeine does temporarily increase alertness, only nutrition, exercise, and rest can give us real energy.

So the next time you're tempted to reach for a caffeinated beverage, consider a brisk walk, a yoga session, or a few minutes of deep breathing instead. Herbs such as Ashwagandha, Rhodiola, and Schizandra can also help promote balanced energy by regulating your body's stress response and supporting your adrenal glands.

If you're not ready to kick the caffeine habit altogether, try drinking green tea instead of coffee or soda. While green tea does contain 30 to 60 mg of caffeine per eight-ounce cup, the stimulating effect is moderated by L-theanine, an amino acid with calming properties. Even better, green tea is one of the richest sources of antioxidant phytochemicals.

LEARN MORE

- *Adaptogens*, David Winston
- *Energy Addict*, Jon Gordon

"The goal of life is to make your heartbeat match the beat of the universe, to match your nature with Nature."

JOSEPH CAMPBELL

9 Listen to Your Heart.

If you exercise regularly but don't feel you're making much progress, the best approach is not necessarily to step up the intensity. In fact, lackluster results could mean that you need to slow down your pace. Excessive tiredness after exercise is another clue that you may be pushing yourself too hard.

The best way to tell whether you're exercising in your aerobic range is to measure your heart rate. That's why a heart rate monitor is one of the most useful pieces of exercise equipment you can buy. You'll also need to calculate your target heart rate. While no heart rate formula is infallible, Dr. Phillip Maffetone's 180 Formula is a good place to start:

1. First, *subtract your age from 180.*
2. Second, modify this number depending on your physical condition:
    a. If you have had a major illness or you take any regular medication, *subtract 10.*
    b. If have been exercising, but you've been injured, you aren't improving, or if you often suffer from colds, flu, or allergies, *subtract 5.*
    c. If you have been exercising at least four times a week without any injury, and you don't get colds or flu more than a few times a year, *do nothing.*
    d. If you have been exercising for more than two years without injury, you have been making progress, and you are a competitive athlete, *add 5.*
3. The resulting number is your Maximum Aerobic Heart Rate (MAHR). The upper limit of your target heart range is the same as your MAHR. To calculate the lower limit, *subtract 10 from your MAHR.* To ensure that you're exercising aerobically, try to keep your heart rate within this ten-point range.

Learn More

◆ *In Fitness and In Health*, Phillip B. Maffetone

Energize **51**

"An early-morning walk is a blessing for the whole day."

HENRY DAVID THOREAU

10 Begin the Journey of 10,000 Steps.

Of all the exercises you could do, walking is one of the simplest and most versatile. If you haven't been physically active, walking is easy to ease into. If you're already in good shape, you can still get a good workout by stepping up the pace. And while you may find it hard to fit an hour of exercise into your schedule, a few minutes of walking here and there can add up to a significant increase in your activity level.

Leonardo DaVinci envisioned the pedometer, and Thomas Jefferson created the first working model. It wasn't until the 1960s, however, that the humble gadget became widely popular. It happened in Japan, where *Manpo-kei* ("ten thousand steps meter") started out as a marketing slogan and quickly became a movement as millions of Japanese began striving to accumulate 10,000 steps per day. (Most adults take 5,000 to 6,000 steps per day without trying. An additional 4,000 to 5,000 steps is roughly equivalent to 40 minutes of moderate activity.)

Once you have a pedometer to help you monitor your progress, there are lots of ways you can increase your daily step count:
- Instead of grabbing an energy drink, start the day with a brisk walk.
- Burn off stress after work by taking a walk with a friend.
- Grab an empty parking space farther away from the store instead of fighting for a spot close to the entrance.
- Take the stairs instead of the elevator.
- Instead of watching TV, listen to an audiobook while you move. Your body will thank you for it.

Learn More

◆ *The Complete Guide to Walking,* Mark Fenton
➤ *ConsumerSearch Pedometer Reviews* (www.consumersearch.com/pedometers)

Energize **53**

> "Take care of your body. It's the only place you have to live."
>
> — Jim Rohn

Purify

Fig. 7 Activated Carbon and Reverse Osmosis Filters Compared

Contaminant	Activated Carbon	Reverse Osmosis (with Carbon Prefilter)
Chlorine	Removed	Removed
Fluoride	Not removed	Removed
Bacteria	Probably removed	Removed
Parasites	Removed	Removed
Pesticides	Removed	Removed
Solvents	Removed	Removed
Heavy Metals	Possibly Removed	Removed

1 Filter It.

Water purification systems aren't sexy, but one could save you money while protecting you and your family from pollution. In the United States, drinking water has been found to contain over 1,100 potentially toxic compounds. Concerns about the purity of tap water have led to a boom in bottled water sales. But bottled water isn't always free of contaminants, either—a 1999 study conducted by the National Resources Defense Council found that a third of bottled waters were contaminated with chemicals or bacteria.

Compared with the alternatives, a home filtration system is the most convenient, cost effective, and environmentally conscious way to ensure a supply of safe, great-tasting drinking water. The two main types of water filter on the market are *activated carbon* and *reverse osmosis*. Which one is best for you will depend on your budget and priorities.

Activated carbon filters are inexpensive and they work fast, guaranteeing that you always have water when you need it. Some are even sufficiently compact to be taken along when you travel. This type of filter removes chlorine, parasites, pesticides, solvents, most bacteria, and possibly some heavy metals.

In addition to being more expensive than activated carbon filters, reverse osmosis systems are bulky, and they typically need to be installed under your sink. The advantage of a reverse osmosis filter is that it removes fluoride and heavy metals, in addition to all the contaminants removed by an activated carbon filter.

Learn More

◆ *The Drinking Water Book*, Colin Ingram
▸ *ConsumerSearch Water Filter Reviews* (www.consumersearch.com/water-filters)

Fig. 8 Soft Drinks by the Numbers

1 The United States leads the world in soft drink consumption. (The other countries in the top five are Ireland, Canada, Norway, and Belgium.)

2.5 The average American's caloric intake from soft drinks and fruit drinks more than doubled between 1977 and 2001, reaching 7 percent of total calories.

20 The average American consumes 20 percent of his or her calories in the form of sugar, of which soft drinks are a major source.

41 The average person consumes 41 ounces of liquids each day, including coffee, tea, fruit juice, and soft drinks.

60 According to a 2001 study, schoolchildren who consumed just one soft drink per day were 60 percent more likely to become obese.

500 One soft drink may contain up to 500 mg of phosphorus, but virtually no calcium. Some authorities believe that this imbalance has contributed to the high rate of osteoporosis in the United States.

2 Don't Be a Softie.

The soft drink has become America's beverage of choice, relegating water to the position of backbencher. Today, more than forty percent of Americans drink no more than two glasses of water per day, and twenty percent don't drink water at all.

But just because we can choose from a bewildering variety of sweet, caffeinated beverages doesn't mean we should. In addition to being the number one source of calories in the American diet, soft drinks promote diabetes by keeping our blood sugar levels elevated. Many soft drinks are also high in caffeine and phosphorus, both of which may contribute to osteoporosis if consumed in excessive amounts.

The problem isn't limited to soft drinks, however. Coffee drinks, energy drinks, and sugar-enriched fruit drinks are all best thought of as liquid candy—okay as an occasional treat, but not as our standard-issue thirst-quencher. And while fruit juice can be a good source of vitamins and antioxidants, whole fruit is a better choice. Fruit juice gives you all the calories of whole fruit, but with none of the fiber.

As for sports drinks, they're rarely necessary. After an hour or more of strenuous exercise, you can replace your electrolytes by adding ¼ teaspoon of salt to a quart of water. But if a brisk walk or thirty minutes of aerobics is the extent of your workout, good old-fashioned water is all you need.

Learn More

- *Soft Drinks and Health* (www.cspinet.org/sodapop)
- *Soft Drinks: America's Other Drinking Problem* (www.westonaprice.org/modernfood/soft.html)

"I believe that water is the only drink for a wise man."

HENRY DAVID THOREAU

3 A Better Bottle.

After you've gone to the trouble of filtering your water, why carry it around in a plastic bottle that may be hazardous to your health? Polycarbonate, the material used in the construction of most plastic water bottles, contains a substance called bisphenol-A (BPA). Unfortunately, some of this chemical can leach into our water, and studies have linked BPA exposure to increased risk for a number of serious diseases, including breast and prostate cancer, heart disease, diabetes, and liver abnormalities. Because of BPA's potential to disrupt normal development, it is of particular concern for pregnant women, newborns, and young children.

In response to concerns about BPA, health-savvy consumers have started ditching their polycarbonate bottles in favor of stainless steel. An alloy containing iron, carbon, chromium, and sometimes nickel, stainless steel is highly durable, resistant to corrosion, and nonreactive, which is why it's often used for food- and medical-grade equipment. But not all steel bottles are created equal—some are lined with polycarbonate, presenting the same health risks as a plastic bottle.

Bilt™ and Klean Kanteen™ are two companies that make handsome stainless steel bottles without plastic liners. Both companies also use lids made from polypropylene, a food-grade plastic that does not contain BPA.

Learn More

▸ *Bilt* (www.bilt.ca)
▸ *Klean Kanteen* (www.kleankanteen.com)

"Smile, breathe,
and go slowly."

Thich Nhat Hanh

4 Just Breathe.

For something we do every minute of every day, breathing is easy to take for granted. The concept of breathing exercises can even seem silly—the fact that we're alive, you might say, means that we're already breathing fine. Yet perhaps there is a reason that breathing meditations are an important part of many venerable spiritual traditions.

In Hinduism, proper breathing is integral to Hatha yoga. Buddhists practice *Anapanasati*, or "mindfulness of breathing," to quiet the mind and ultimately attain enlightenment. Taoists have long believed that breathing meditation strengthens the *chi*, improves physical health, and even aids the pursuit of immortality.

On a less-lofty level, scientific studies have shown many benefits of breathing meditation, including greater productivity, less stress, lower blood pressure, and a reduction in the need for medical care.

There are thousands of different meditation techniques, none of which is necessarily more correct than any other. Experiment with different methods until you find the one that works best for you. A good place to start is by sitting comfortably, either in a chair or on the floor with your head and back straight. Close your eyes and breathe slowly through your nose. Now concentrate on your breath. If your mind wanders—and it will!—gently return your focus to your breath. Try to maintain this gentle focus for five to ten minutes, eventually working up to longer sessions.

Learn More

◆ *Free Your Breath, Free Your Life*, Dennis Lewis
➤ *Learning Meditation* (www.learningmeditation.com)

"I know that our bodies were made to thrive only in pure air, and the scenes in which pure air is found."

JOHN MUIR

5 Filter It, Redux.

When you think about air pollution, do you picture smoggy skylines and freeways clogged with cars? Then you may be surprised to learn that the biggest air quality threats are inside our homes and offices. In fact, the EPA reports that indoor levels of some pollutants are two to five times higher than outdoor levels. Indoor air quality is particularly important because we spend ninety percent of our time indoors—and more than half of that time inside our homes.

Part of the problem is the widespread use of potentially toxic chemicals; in addition to mold, bacteria, and allergens, the typical home may harbor as many as 1,500 hazardous compounds. Poor air quality is also to some extent an unintended consequence of our push for greater energy efficiency. By installing insulation and patching the leaks around doors and windows, we have reduced the flow of outside air and increased the concentration of indoor pollutants.

Here are five simple ways to improve your indoor air quality:
- Avoid adding to the problem by using natural products whenever possible.
- Improve ventilation by opening the windows on pleasant days.
- Consider a HEPA air filtration system, which effectively removes dust, dander, pollen, and mold.
- Have your home tested for radon.
- Make sure your gas furnace and appliances are functioning properly.

Learn More

◆ *The Healthy Home*, Linda Mason Hunter
➤ *ConsumerSearch Air Purifier Reviews*
(www.consumersearch.com/air-purifiers)

"The body is your temple. Keep it pure and clean for the soul to reside in."

B.K.S. Iyengar

6 Spring Clean.

Thousands of years ago, the only contaminants that most people had to worry about were viral and bacterial pathogens. Metal toxicity was an unlikely concern, and the whole range of artificial organic compounds simply hadn't been invented yet.

Today, we are exposed to toxins every day. They're in the air we breathe, the food we eat, and some of the substances that come in contact with our skin. Many of us also use drugs—whether prescription, over-the-counter, or recreational—that can have harmful effects on the human body.

Some people attempt to detoxify with water or juice fasting, but these methods aren't for everyone. Fasting can lead to fatigue or malnutrition, especially in people who are already undernourished. A gentler way to help your body eliminate toxins is to spend a few weeks on a detox diet.

This type of diet involves eliminating those foods that are frequently harmful (sugar, caffeine, alcohol) or that tend to promote congestion (meats, dairy products, fats and oils, nuts). Instead, emphasize foods that are rich in fiber and nutrients, such as fresh fruits and vegetables, fruit and vegetable juices, and whole grains. You can also include sprouted legumes and raw or sprouted seeds, and be sure to drink plenty of fresh water.

LEARN MORE

◆ *The Detox Book,* Bruce Fife
◆ *The New Detox Diet,* Elson Haas and Daniella Chace

Fig. 9   The Electromagnetic Spectrum

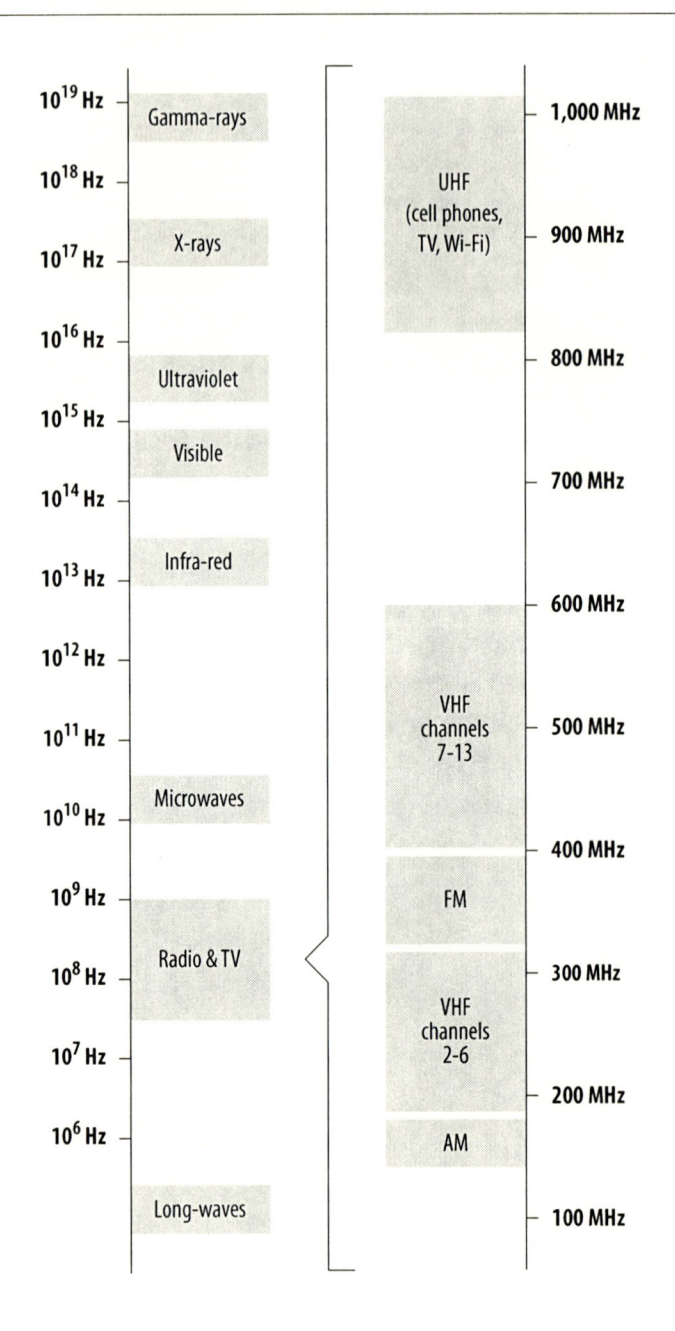

10^{19} Hz	Gamma-rays		1,000 MHz
10^{18} Hz		UHF (cell phones, TV, Wi-Fi)	
10^{17} Hz	X-rays		900 MHz
10^{16} Hz			800 MHz
	Ultraviolet		
10^{15} Hz	Visible		
10^{14} Hz			700 MHz
10^{13} Hz	Infra-red		
			600 MHz
10^{12} Hz			
10^{11} Hz		VHF channels 7-13	500 MHz
10^{10} Hz	Microwaves		400 MHz
10^{9} Hz		FM	
10^{8} Hz	Radio & TV		300 MHz
10^{7} Hz		VHF channels 2-6	200 MHz
10^{6} Hz		AM	
	Long-waves		100 MHz

7 Catch That E.L.F.

As you read these words, invisible waves of information are all around you. There are FM radio signals encoded for pop music, and TV signals carrying local news programs. At a higher frequency, in the crowded UHF band, cell phones and wireless networking devices transmit their data. And all along the spectrum is the electromagnetic noise produced by electric wiring, appliances, and fluorescent lights.

Some people blame electromagnetic radiation for causing symptoms such as headaches, dizziness, and sleep disturbances. In the laboratory, researchers have altered cells by exposing them to very strong electromagnetic fields. Research into the real-world health effects of electromagnetic exposure has yielded mixed results, with some, but not all, studies showing increased risk of cancer.

To eliminate all electromagnetic radiation would be virtually impossible, but you can reduce your exposure through a few simple techniques:

- Remove all plugged-in devices from your bedroom, or at least from the area around your bed.
- Avoid placing the head of your bed against a wall that has an appliance, fuse box, TV, or computer on the other side.
- Throw out your electric blanket.
- If you think electromagnetic fields might be affecting your sleep, use your fusebox to shut off all power to your bedroom at night.

Learn More

◆ *Electromagnetic Fields*, B. Blake Levitt
◆ *Healthy Living Spaces*, Daniel P. Stih

Fig. 10 Commonly Allergic Foods

Meats and Poultry

Beef	Chicken	

Fish and Seafood

All fish and shellfish

Eggs and Dairy

Eggs	All dairy foods	

Grains

Barley	Corn	Oats
Rye	Wheat	

Legumes

Peanuts	Soy	

Nuts and Seeds

All nuts

Fruits and Vegetables

Citrus fruit and juice	Corn	Tomatoes

Other

Alcohol	Artificial additives	Caffeine
Chocolate	Sugar	

8 Take a Food Holiday.

Is there a food you just have to have? Your cravings may be caused by an addiction, which is often the result of a food allergy or sensitivity. An elimination diet is a simple and inexpensive way to test for food allergies—simple, but not easy, because temporarily giving up your favorite foods is an exercise in self-discipline.

This type of diet involves removing commonly allergic foods from your diet for a two-week period, then slowly reintroducing them. Keep a journal, noting how you feel before, immediately after, and several hours after reintroducing a suspect food. Adding back one food per day will make it easier to tell which foods are causing allergic symptoms. If you have a reaction to a particular food, you can reduce, rotate, or eliminate it from your diet entirely.

See the facing page for a list of commonly allergic foods, and remember to watch out for hidden ingredients—foods such as wheat, corn, soy, dairy, and sugar are nearly ubiquitous in processed foods. Eating whole foods will make it easier to eliminate common allergens from your diet.

Learn More

◆ *The Allergy Exclusion Diet*, Jill Carter and Alison Edwards
◆ *Food Allergies and Food Intolerance*, Jonathan Brostoff and Linda Gamlin

"There is a sufficiency in the world for man's need but not for man's greed."

Mohandas K. Gandhi

9 Clean Up Your Act.

If you're like most people, your family's health is one of your most important reasons for keeping your house clean. Ironically, however, there are toxic chemicals in many of the products we use to keep our dishes sparkling, our floors polished, and our drains unclogged. Some of these hazardous substances are absorbed through our skin; others are vaporized into the air, adding to indoor pollution. And they don't just disappear when we flush them down the sink—instead, they may end up contaminating our groundwater, lakes, and oceans.

Fortunately, it's easy to make the switch to green cleaning supplies. Check out a natural foods store for a wide selection of natural products. Or go retro and make your own cleaning supplies from ingredients you already have around the house:

- Replace commercial abrasive cleansers with baking soda.
- Use lemon juice to dissolve soap scum and hard water deposits. (You can also use lemon juice to shine brass and copper.)
- Make your own furniture polish by thoroughly mixing one cup of olive oil with ½ cup lemon juice.
- Make an effective all-purpose cleaner by mixing equal parts water and white vinegar. It's safe, cheap, and won't harm most surfaces (but don't use it on marble).

Learn More

◆ *Better Basics for the Home*, Annie Berthold-Bond
◆ *Organic Housekeeping*, Ellen Sandbeck

"Taking joy in living is a woman's best cosmetic."

Rosalind Russell

10 Discover Natural Beauty.

That pesky blemish may not be the only thing your concealer is hiding. Many cosmetics contain chemicals such as acrylamide, formaldehyde, and ethylene oxide, all of which are on the EPA's list of known carcinogens. Could these substances pose a danger to your health? The cosmetics industry says no, yet human skin is highly permeable—that's why transdermal patches are an effective delivery method for many medications.

The FDA doesn't review new cosmetics before they come to market. Nor does the agency have the power to recall cosmetics that have proved to be harmful. Can we depend on the cosmetics industry to regulate itself? And why take any risk when natural alternatives are readily available?

Visit your natural foods store for a selection of chemical-free cosmetics and hair care products. If you don't have a natural foods store in your area, visit AllNaturalCosmetics.com for a variety of natural cosmetics and personal care products made without mineral oil, solvents, or artificial colorings. Selected products are also certified as organic, vegan, gluten-free, fragrance-free, and low-fragrance.

If you're feeling especially adventurous, check out *Organic Body Care Recipes*, a book that tells you how to make your own cosmetics from herbs, spices, essential oils, and other natural ingredients that you can buy at the grocery store or grow in your own garden.

Learn More

◆ *The Green Beauty Guide*, Julie Gabriel
◆ *Organic Body Care Recipes*, Stephanie Tourles
▸ *AllNaturalCosmetics.com* (www.allnaturalcosmetics.com)

> *"Simplicity is the ultimate sophistication."*
>
> Leonardo Da Vinci

Simplify

"The wisdom of life consists in the elimination of non-essentials."

LIN YUTANG

1 Simplify Your Schedule.

Life may be a banquet, but are your eyes bigger than your stomach? In a world that seems to offer endless possibilities, most of us are intent on getting as much as we can out of life. But this admirable impulse can lead us to take on too many commitments. In our zeal to live life fully, we end up feeling overwhelmed. In our fear of missing out on anything, we find ourselves too busy to give our full attention to anything.

We also overschedule ourselves because we're afraid of disappointing someone else, whether it's the boss who wants us to work overtime or the friend who wants us to campaign for her favorite cause.

But while our options are infinite, our time is a non-renewable resource. Each day gives you just twenty-four hours, and chances are you've already filled them up with something. This means that every time you say yes to a new commitment, you need to say no to something else.

To decide what to give up, use the 80/20 rule: Twenty percent of the things you do are responsible for eighty percent of the results. Learn to separate the essential from the trivial. Ask yourself, "Which activities really pay the bills? Which ones help me grow? Which ones bring me the most joy?"

If we always say yes to other people, we're probably saying no to our own needs. When we learn to say no more consciously, we begin to value ourselves as highly as we deserve.

Learn More

◆ *Find More Time*, Laura Stack
◆ *Simplify Your Time*, Marcia Ramsland

*"Concentration is
the secret of strength."*

RALPH WALDO EMERSON

2 SINGLETASK.

You're eating breakfast, checking your hair in the mirror, talking on the phone, and adjusting the volume on the radio at the same time. Then you glance at a road sign and realize you've missed your exit. When it comes to multitasking, you can give a fourteen-year-old a run for his money. But have you thought about the price you pay for multitasking? And does it really make you more productive?

In a very real sense, multitasking is an illusion. Scientists have found that our minds are really only capable of focusing on one thing at a time. When we think we're multitasking, we're actually switching back and forth between different tasks so rapidly that we feel like we're doing ten things at once. By preventing us from giving anything our full attention, multitasking adds to our sense that we never have enough time. It increases our risk of errors, with some studies finding that using a cell phone while driving is as dangerous as driving drunk. And multitasking can actually reduce our efficiency by forcing us to switch gears every time we change from one task to another and back again.

To start breaking the multitasking addiction, decide on your most important priority, then give it your full attention until it's finished. If you get distracted, take a quick rest break instead of surfing the web. Check your email no more than once or twice a day, answering all important emails immediately, and filing or deleting the rest. Use the same approach to manage your voicemail, and enjoy your new sense of focus.

LEARN MORE

◆ *The Myth of Multitasking*, Dave Crenshaw
◆ *The Practicing Mind*, Thomas M. Sterner

"The flood of print has turned reading into a process of gulping rather than savoring."

WARREN CHAPPELL

3 Go on a Media Diet.

Before the invention of the printing press, few people owned even a single book. Today, Google puts over a trillion pages at our fingertips, and the Sunday edition of the *New York Times* contains more words than an educated eighteenth-century European read during his or her entire lifetime. The average American consumes 3,000 advertising messages per day, a sixfold increase since the early 1970s. The average corporate employee communicates nearly two hundred times a day by phone, fax, and email.

Today, our biggest problem isn't a lack of information, but an information glut. Extraneous information wastes time and distracts us from the things that really matter. According to some psychologists, a surfeit of information can even lead to sleeping problems, difficulty concentrating, and lowered immune function.

We consume some forms of media because they're entertaining, and others because we think they're important. To cut back on our media consumption, we can spend more time engaging in active recreation rather than passively watching TV. As for the newspapers and TV shows we "need" to watch, how much news is really important, and how much is media hype?

In addition to newspapers and magazines, pay attention to your consumption of TV and radio programs, blogs, and podcasts. And when you really want to get away from it all, spend a three-day weekend with your computer and phone turned off. It's cheaper than a cruise, and surprisingly restorative.

LEARN MORE

◆ *The Four-Hour Work Week,* Timothy Ferriss
◆ *TechnoStress,* Michelle M. Weil and Larry D. Rosen

"True silence is the rest of the mind; it is to the spirit what sleep is to the body, nourishment and refreshment."

WILLIAM PENN

4 Lower the Volume.

Can't hear yourself think? Blame the ubiquity of motor vehicles, power tools, and beeping, buzzing, whistling, and whirring devices of all kinds. In moments of irritation, it's easy to sympathize with the protagonist of the 2007 film *Noise*, a lawyer who becomes an anti-noise vigilante and ultimately loses his job, his marriage, and his apartment to his quixotic crusade against blaring car alarms.

As irritating as it is, however, noise is more than just an annoyance. Hearing loss, which audiologists once believed to be a normal aspect of aging, is actually an avoidable consequence of our noisy modern environment. Noise interferes with sleep and suppresses immune function. Prolonged exposure triggers a stress response, leading in turn to higher levels of adrenaline and cortisol, higher blood pressure, and even increased risk of a heart attack.

While it's impossible to eliminate noise from your life entirely, you can take steps to reduce its impact:

- Take noise levels into consideration the next time you're shopping for yard equipment, a home appliance, or a personal computer.
- Befriend your neighbors so that they're more likely to cooperate if a noise problem occurs.
- Learn the noise abatement laws in your city. If you think a violation is occurring, you can help make your case with a sound level meter (you can get one at RadioShack for less than $50).
- At home and on the go, make life a little quieter with a pair of noise-cancelling headphones, which actively block out background noise, but not your favorite music.

Learn More

▸ *Quiet Gadgets and Products* (www.quiet.org/gadgets.htm)
▸ *NoiseOFF* (www.noiseoff.org)

"I don't believe in email. I'm an old-fashioned girl. I prefer calling and hanging up."

SARAH JESSICA PARKER

5 Unsubscribe.

Each year, the average American receives over 700 telemarketing calls, around 2,200 junk e-mails, and 41 pounds of junk mail. You can save time, eliminate distractions, and help the environment by reducing your exposure to commercial messages.

The quickest way to cut down on telemarketing calls is to add your number to the National Do Not Call Registry. When salespeople call, you can also ask them to permanently remove you from their calling lists. If the same company calls you again, report them to the Federal Trade Commission via the Do Not Call website.

Dropping out of society may be the only way to escape direct mail altogether, but you can reduce it by not giving out your contact information unnecessarily. Get an unlisted number, and stop mailing in product registration cards—you're usually covered by the warranty as long as you keep the receipt. To get off the mailing lists you're already on, you may need to contact a number of different companies and organizations—see Privacy Rights Clearinghouse's Junk Mail Factsheet for a solid list.

Legitimate Internet marketers are legally required to let you unsubscribe from their email lists, either by clicking a link or sending an email. Unfortunately, spammers don't care about such niceties. To cut down on spam, give your email address only to people you trust, and use a free disposable email address (such as Mailinator) when you register for websites.

Learn More

- *Junk Mail Factsheet* (www.privacyrights.org/fs/fs4-junk.htm)
- *Mailinator* (www.mailinator.com)
- *National Do Not Call Registry* (www.donotcall.gov)

"When you realize there is nothing lacking, the whole world belongs to you."

Lao Tzu

6 CAN THE CLUTTER.

You don't have to practice *fung shui* to believe that a clean, well-organized environment promotes peace of mind. Even better, cleaning experts say that reducing clutter can cut housework by forty percent. Here are some suggestions to get you started:

- *Be persistent.* Don't try to conquer years' worth of accumulated clutter in a single bout. Instead, commit to organizing your house for fifteen minutes a day.
- *Take one room at a time.* Declutter your home room by room, closet by closet. Getting one room fully organized will motivate you to tackle the next one.
- *Use the three-box method to overcome indecision.* Label the first two boxes "Keep" and "Give Away." The third "box" is a trash can.
- *Give it a year.* You know those things you don't use, but think you might use "someday?" Put them in a box, seal it, and date it for a year from now. If you haven't opened the box in a year, give it away without opening it.
- *Stop clutter before it starts.* Stop bringing new stuff into your home. Or follow the one-in, two-out rule—for every item that enters your home, get rid of two things you already have.
- *Share more, spend less.* Before you buy that book or DVD, check to see if your local library has a copy. And instead of buying a power tool you'll only use twice a year, think about renting it or borrowing it from a neighbor.

LEARN MORE

◆ *The Clutter Cure*, Judi Culbertson
➤ *OrganizedHome* (www.organizedhome.com)

"You give but little when you give of your possessions. It is when you give of yourself that you truly give."

KAHLIL GIBRAN

7 Give from the Heart.

They say it's better to give than to receive, but don't tell that to the harried last-minute shopper. Here are five ways to make gift-giving easier, less expensive, more meaningful, and gentler on the environment:

- *Buy one gift for everyone.* If you participate in a Secret Santa gift exchange at work, you already know how this concept works. You may not think your extended family would go for the same idea, but you'll never know unless you ask. They may share your desire to make gift-giving dramatically simpler.
- *Do it yourself.* If you're handy with a needle, you can knit scarves, throws, or blankets. If you're talented in the kitchen, indulge your friends and family with homemade goodies. You could also compile a book of family recipes, edit the best of your home movies onto a DVD, or build a website chronicling a special friendship.
- *Buy intangibles.* Intangible gifts don't have to be wrapped or shipped, and they won't contribute to the recipient's clutter crisis. Buy someone a theater or zoo membership, a certificate for a massage or manicure, or adopt an endangered animal in his or her name.
- *Give the gift of life.* Be unique and honor the environment at the same time. Choose a living gift such as a house plant, a collection of seed packets, or a potted tree that can be planted in the yard come springtime.
- *It's a wrap.* Reuse wrapping paper, or wrap your presents in old maps, newspaper comics pages, or scraps of fabric or tissue paper left over from craft projects.

Learn More

▶ *SecretSanta.com* (www.secretsanta.com)
▶ *Treehugger Holiday Gift Guide* (www.treehugger.com/giftguide)

"He who cannot forgive breaks the bridge over which he himself must pass."

GEORGE HERBERT

8 Let Go.

Your closets may be as neat as a pin, but you can't achieve simplicity if your mental living space is crowded with thoughts that no longer serve a purpose in your life.

To reduce your mental clutter, start by examining your ideas about what you can and cannot control. Our stress levels are reduced when we have a healthy sense of control over our lives, but increased by trying to control the uncontrollable. Among the things that we can't control (but often try to) are other people's thoughts and actions, everything that has happened in the past, and much that will happen in the future.

It's important to take responsibility for your choices, but it's a waste of energy to dwell on memories that you associate with guilt, regret, or self-recrimination. Try to approach your mistakes with scientific detachment, examining them for useful data and letting go of negative emotions.

After you've forgiven yourself, think of other people toward whom you harbor anger or resentment. Many psychological theories advise us to analyze our negative emotions, but recent studies suggest that ruminating on past traumas is more likely to cause a deepening of negative emotions than genuine healing. We sometimes cling to resentments because we feel that those who have harmed us don't deserve to be forgiven. Usually, however, those people aren't even aware of our anger, and we're the ones who suffer. Forgiveness is less a gift that we give to others than it is a gift we give to ourselves.

Learn More

◆ *Forgiveness Is a Choice*, Robert D. Enright
➤ *The Forgiveness Project* (www.theforgivenessproject.com)

"He who would travel happily must travel light."

ANTOINE DE SAINT-EXUPERY

9 Travel Light.

Do you ever have to remind yourself that vacations are supposed to be fun? Here are six ways to make your next trip easier and more affordable:

- *Do your homework.* Instead of paying for a guided tour, use a guidebook and the Internet to find free or inexpensive attractions ahead of time.
- *Pack light.* Start with the essentials and ruthlessly eliminate anything that won't fit into one backpack and a carry-on suitcase. Bring a change of clothes and a good book, but why bother packing shampoo when you can buy it at your destination?
- *Get there for less.* Many budget airlines don't show up on travel sites, but you can find them on Attitudetravel.com. Book your flight in advance, and be flexible about your travel dates. You can often save even more money by purchasing your ticket outside the U.S. Pick a destination with good public transportation, and you won't have to rent a car once you get there.
- *Sleep outside the box.* Instead of staying at a pricey hotel, try a hostel or home exchange. Despite their image as youth-oriented dorms, many hostels offer private rooms.
- *Stay closer to home.* You'll save on travel expenses by driving your own car, and you may also pay less for food and accommodations if you avoid popular destinations.
- *Don't leave home at all.* Make it known that you'll be incommunicado for the weekend, then play tourist in an area of your city that you don't normally visit.

Learn More

◆ *Travel Light*, Joy Nyquist
↖ *Attitude Travel* (www.attitudetravel.com)

"Christmas is not as much about opening our presents as opening our hearts."

JANICE MAEDITERE

10 CELEBRATE SIMPLY.

RECIPE FOR HOLIDAY STRESS
Combine one dozen relatives under a single roof. Add simmering resentments and a splash of eggnog. Fold in time pressures, financial anxieties, and unrealistic expectations. Stew for two weeks. Serves 12.

If this recipe rings a bell, you may want to try some new ingredients this holiday season:
- *Acknowledge your feelings.* If you're feeling anxious, lonely, or depressed, talk to someone who's going through the same thing.
- *Be realistic.* When we expect the holidays to be like a Frank Capra movie, we set ourselves up for disappointment. Instead of expecting interpersonal conflicts to be resolved, focus on setting them aside until the holidays are over.
- *Set limits.* You can enjoy the holidays without jeopardizing your health and financial wellbeing. Splurge a little, but without overindulging in food and drink. Show others you appreciate them, but without throwing your budget out the window.
- *Don't try to do it all.* If you're always the one who gets stuck doing the cooking, cleaning, shopping, and wrapping, start delegating some tasks to other family members.
- *Decommercialize.* Instead of running up a big tab at the mall, celebrate with less expensive but more meaningful activities, such as baking cookies, caroling, volunteering, giving to needy families, and spending time outdoors.

LEARN MORE

◆ *Simple Pleasures for the Holidays*, Susannah Seton

"Renew thyself completely each day; do it again, and again, and forever again."

CHINESE INSCRIPTION CITED BY HENRY DAVID THOREAU

Renew

"Anything done with focus, awareness or mindfulness is a meditation."

DAVID HARP

1 Go with the Flow.

Psychologists call it flow. Buddhists call it mindfulness. Athletes call it "being in the zone." Whatever term you use, it's what happens when you become so absorbed in an activity that you lose track of time. The outside world seems to disappear, as do your worries about the future and that bothersome twinge in your knee. It's the state that artists and scientists experience during their moments of greatest creativity. But you don't have to be Leonardo da Vinci to experience flow in your own life.

People find flow in many activities, including reading, dancing, painting, writing, bridge, and soccer. Despite the outward dissimilarities, activities that induce flow have several things in common.

First, they need to be difficult enough to be challenging, but not so difficult that they're beyond your capabilities. Take tennis, for example. You also have a clear goal (getting the ball over the net) and a sense of control (you're the one holding the racket). When you act, you receive immediate feedback (whether you ace the ball into your opponent's ad court or lodge it in a nearby tree.)

Mihaly Csikszentmihalyi, a researcher with a tongue-twister of a name (it's pronounced me-HIGH cheeks-sent-me-high-EE), has found that people who regularly experience flow are psychologically healthier than those who immerse themselves in passive entertainment. Translation: Turn off the TV and go do something that stimulates your mind. It seems your mom was right all along.

Learn More

◆ *Flow: The Psychology of Optimal Experience*, Mihaly Csikszentmihalyi
◆ *Zen and the Art of Happiness*, Chris Prentiss

> "The greatest gift of the garden is the restoration of the five senses."

HANNA RION

2 Bring Nature Home.

To our ancestors, nature was an elemental force, by turns nourishing and deadly. Today, cocooned as we are by layers of technology, it's easy for us to forget how thoroughly we still depend upon the natural world. Yet a growing body of research suggests that nature—in addition to providing the air we breathe and the food we eat—may also be vital to our psychological health. In fact, over a hundred studies have found that the natural world is a powerful antidote to stress.

Fortunately, nature exists in suburban backyards as well as untamed wilderness, and even those of us who live in the big city can spend more time in nature. Here are just five of the many ways you can bring nature home:

- *Plant a native garden.* Consider giving top priority to plants that attract butterflies, hummingbirds, and other colorful visitors.
- *Provide water.* Buy a birdbath or basin, and change the water regularly.
- *Provide food.* Hang birdfeeders within sight of your windows. Attract a variety of species by offering more than one type of food.
- *Provide shelter.* Leave leaf litter alone, and add a few rocks and logs.
- *Cultivate awareness.* Keep a camera handy, and write about your discoveries in a nature journal.

Learn More

◆ *Bringing Nature Home*, Douglas W. Tallamy
◆ *Keeping a Nature Journal*, Clare W. Leslie and Charles E. Roth
◆ *Sharing Nature with Children*, Joseph B. Cornell
▸ Create a Certified Wildlife Habitat (www.nwf.org/backyard)

"Gratitude is the memory of the heart."

Jean Baptiste Massieu

3 Keep a Gratitude Journal.

Between our memories of the past and our worries about the future, it's easy to forget that all we ever really have is the moment we're living right now. Cultivating gratitude can help us focus on the good things in our lives and learn to separate the things we really care about from the things we don't. Studies have also confirmed that keeping a gratitude journal can dramatically increase our levels of happiness and life satisfaction.

Keeping a gratitude journal is easy. Start by purchasing a blank notebook or journal, and begin writing in it every day. Like any new habit, journaling can be hard to remember at first. Keep your journal in a convenient place with a pen close at hand, and make it part of your routine by writing at the same time every evening—perhaps right before you go to bed.

Each day, try to write down at least five things that make you feel glad to be alive. Few of them will be as important as a big promotion or a new car; in fact, one of the best reasons for keeping a gratitude journal is to cultivate appreciation for the small pleasures that can easily go unnoticed: a child's laughter, a perfectly-shaped stone, or the crunch of autumn leaves. Like a reporter always on the lookout for a good story, get in the habit of observing things that inspire gratitude. And if you'd like to share your good feelings with the world, there are several websites designed to let you do just that.

Learn More

- *Thanks!*, Robert Emmons
- *ButterBeeHappy* (www.butterbeehappy.com)
- *Thanks-O-Meter.com* (www.thanks-o-meter.com)

"We visit others as a matter of social obligation. How long has it been since we have visited with ourselves?"

Morris Adler

4 SEEK SOLITUDE.

A lonely person and a solitary one may look the same to an outside observer, yet there's a world of difference in how they feel inside. Neither loneliness nor solitude is synonymous with being alone: It's possible to be alone without being lonely, and equally possible to feel lonely while surrounded by people—you may have felt this way in a crowd of jostling strangers, or worse, at a family dinner when you felt at odds with those you expected to be closest to you.

Solitude, on the other hand, is a positive state of enjoying your own company. Loneliness is an imposition, but solitude is a choice. And while loneliness can be the worst form of punishment, our busy, clamorous world has made solitude a delightful luxury.

Some of us are afraid of solitude, so we fill up our lives with people, sound, and broadcast images in order to avoid spending time alone with our own thoughts. But by doing so, we're missing a great opportunity to reflect on our lives, recharge our creative batteries, and learn how simple it can be to enjoy ourselves.

To change your attitude toward solitude, you can start by changing how you think about other people. Could it be that the amount of time you spend with others is less important than the quality of that time? Then why not spend some time alone, without distractions, and see how good your own company can be. You may find as a result that you become better company for others, too.

LEARN MORE

◆ *Celebrating Time Alone: Stories of Splendid Solitude*, Lionel Fisher
◆ *The Wonders of Solitude*, Dale Salwak

*"In the depth of winter
I finally learned that
within me there lay an
invincible summer."*

Albert Camus

5 Cultivate Optimism.

If you were a cartoon character, would there be a tiny storm cloud constantly hovering over your head? Or are you the kind of person who looks on the sunny side of life? Science suggests that our attitudes are partly shaped by our genes, but not entirely. This means that we can learn to be more optimistic.

Cognitive psychologists believe that the difference between an optimist and a pessimist boils down to how we perceive the *permanence* and *pervasiveness* of the events in our lives. Suppose you have a flat tire on your way to work. If you're an optimist, you see the event as temporary and specific. It's a hassle, but you'll get it fixed. And one bad commute doesn't change all the other good things in your life.

If you're a pessimist, your mind races ahead to the dire repercussions. You'll be late for work, and then your boss will yell at you. What if you get fired and can't pay your mortgage? You perceive the event as permanent (long-lasting) and pervasive (affecting every aspect of your life).

Like any other behavior, optimism isn't something you can acquire overnight. The good news is that you can practice optimism anywhere, and the only tools you need are your mind and a simple concept. This concept is the ABC model, in which *A* stands for an *Action* or event, such as having a flat tire. This leads to *Consequences*, such as feeling angry or depressed. The *B* is there to remind you that, rather than being inevitable, these consequences are the result of your *Beliefs*. It may sound simplistic, but becoming more aware of your thought patterns is a big step toward becoming a more optimistic person.

LEARN MORE

◆ *Learned Optimism*, Martin Seligman

"Enjoy the little things, for one day you may look back and realize they were the big things."

Robert Brault

6 GIVE YOURSELF A TIME OUT.

If you value achievement, life can seem like an endless ladder. First you ascend rung by rung through grade school. Then come four years of college, perhaps followed by two to four years of graduate school. When you enter the workforce, your career is structured the same way, as a series of promotions leading up to the big payoff: retirement.

While it's important to be capable of postponing gratification in order to achieve long-term goals, it's equally important to enjoy life as you go along. Too many people spend their lives striving to reach the top of the career ladder, only to discover that being top dog isn't as satisfying as they anticipated. Or after sacrificing their health to finance a comfortable retirement, they find themselves at a loss now that their days are no longer filled with work. The lesson is that we need to strike a balance between present and future—working to achieve our goals, but also enjoying small gratifications every day.

Perhaps the simplest reward you can give yourself is a compliment when you've done something well. You could also:

- Buy yourself a small luxury, such as premium stationery, gourmet chocolate, or a unusual blend of tea.
- Catch up with a friend you haven't seen in a while.
- Take an aromatic bath.
- Make homemade popcorn and watch an old movie on DVD.
- Take an inexpensive field trip to a museum, park, or beach.
- Spend an entire day without doing anything productive.

LEARN MORE

◆ *The Art of Doing Nothing,* Veronique Vienne and Erica Lennard
▸ *Simple Pleasures* (www.ocf.berkeley.edu/~wrader/pleasures.html)

"Sometimes the most important thing in a whole day is the rest we take between two deep breaths."

Etty Hillesum

7 DESTRESS PROGRESSIVELY.

Progressive muscle relaxation is a simple but powerful stress management technique designed to slow your heart rate, lower your blood pressure, alleviate muscle tension, and calm your mind.

You will need to be lying on a bed or sitting in a comfortable chair. Make yourself as comfortable as possible, if necessary by loosening any constricting clothing and taking off your shoes. This exercise consists of alternately tensing and relaxing specific groups of muscles. It is important to breathe slowly and deeply the entire time.

Begin by tensing the muscles in your hands. Clench your fists. Hold the tension for ten seconds, then relax for ten to fifteen seconds. If you're not sure how long ten seconds is, silently count up by thousands: "One thousand, two thousand," etc.

Next, in succession, tense and relax your biceps, triceps, and shoulders. Turn your head as far as you can to the right, then to the left. Press your chin into your chest. Open your mouth. Extend your tongue. Curl your tongue back toward your throat. Open your eyes wide, then close them tightly. Tense your buttocks, then your thighs. Pull in your stomach, then extend it as far as you can. Extend your toes away from you, then point them back toward your body. Dig your toes into the floor, then bend them up as far as possible. Remember to relax after each step, and skip any part of the exercise that causes pain.

LEARN MORE

◆ *The Relaxation & Stress Reduction Workbook*, Martha Davis, Elizabeth Robbins Eshelman, Matthew McKay, and Patrick Fanning
◆ *Progressive Relaxation & Autogenic Training*, Carolyn McManus

"Your work is to discover your world and then with all your heart give yourself to it."

BUDDHA

8 Discover Your Signature Strengths.

The word "character" has an old-fashioned sound to it. To have character is undoubtedly a responsible thing to do (like eating your vegetables), but it would seem to be a dubious candidate for the secret to happiness. Yet according to experts in the field of positive psychology, using your character strengths on a daily basis is the surest path to a life of meaning and satisfaction—far more so than a high-paying job, a big house, or a car that goes from zero to sixty in 5.8 seconds.

We can think of character as a compass that helps guide us through a sea of confusing choices to a life in accordance with our deepest values. But although character is intensely personal, it has a universal aspect as well. While some values vary with time and place, a cross-cultural analysis found six core values that are embraced by diverse religious and philosophical traditions: wisdom, courage, humanity, justice, temperance, and transcendence. In the VIA Classification of Character Strengths, these six core values are broken down into 24 more-specific strengths, including curiosity and humor.

To begin leading with your strengths, first seek to understand yourself better. Taking the VIA Character Survey is a good place to start, but you can also learn a lot by asking the right questions. For example, if you could only take ten values with you to a desert island, which ones would they be? There's only one more step, but this is a tough one: Practice your signature strengths daily—at work, at play, and in your relationships.

Learn More

◆ *Authentic Happiness*, Martin Seligman
▸ *VIA Institute on Character* (www.viastrengths.org)

> "Most men pursue pleasure with such breathless haste that they hurry past it."

SOREN KIERKEGAARD

9 Savor.

A lingering kiss, a perfect pop song, and a plate of hot chocolate chip cookies are three of the pleasures that make life worthwhile. If only we could experience them all the time, we think, our lives would be wonderful. The problem with pleasures is that we soon become habituated to them. So while the first taste of chocolate chip cookie moves us to raptures, each subsequent bite is a little less enjoyable. By the time we get down to the crumbs, we're just eating out of habit.

The key to avoiding habituation is to space out your pleasures. You'll enjoy yourself more if you eat a cookie a day for a whole month than if you eat thirty cookies in one sitting. You can also avoid habituation by making a pact with a friend or spouse to surprise each other with things or activities that you each enjoy.

When you do indulge in a pleasure, allow yourself to savor it. Instead of eating in front of the TV, slow down and become completely absorbed in the experience. This means blocking out distracting thoughts as well as distracting sights and sounds.

Whether you're visiting Machu Picchu or just meeting a friend for lunch, taking a photo or souvenir will remind you of the experience later and give you something to reminisce about with others. Sharing your experience—whether at the time, or later, in retelling—is another important way to make it more meaningful. Finally, the moment you reach the top of Mount Everest (or finish a 5K) is not the time for modesty—it's the time to leap, shout, and experience your personal triumph as fully as possible.

Learn More

◆ *Savoring: A New Model of Positive Experience,* Fred B. Bryant and Joseph Veroff

"A generous heart, kind speech, and a life of service and compassion are the things which renew humanity."

BUDDHA

10 Renew Your Spirit.

Religious beliefs come in a bewildering variety of guises. Is it possible to say anything about spirituality that applies to people of all faiths as well as those who don't identify with a religious tradition at all? Every spiritual tradition is unique, yet there are at least four common elements which collectively point the way to a more meaningful life:

- *Connection.* A large part of spirituality is being part of or experiencing a relationship with something larger than oneself. Depending on your beliefs, this "something" may be the natural world, a personal God, or an impersonal force such as the *Tao*.
- *Service.* When we connect with something beyond ourselves, we begin to temper our selfish concerns with responsibility for others. Our enlarged sense of purpose may take the form of serving God, making the world a better place for future generations, or protecting the many species with whom we share our fragile planet.
- *Mindfulness.* Many spiritual practices, including meditation, mantras, and prayer, help to quiet mental chatter and clear the space we need to transcend our everyday concerns. To be mindful is to slow down and pay attention to the moment, without making judgments or imposing our own preconceptions.
- *Hope.* When we surrender responsibility for the things we cannot control and embrace life with confidence, we feel that, as much as appearances might indicate otherwise, *we are safe and all is well.*

Learn More

◆ *Essential Spirituality*, Roger Walsh

Get a Free Coaching Call with the Author of *Everyday Wellness*

I wrote this book to help you **prevent chronic disease and achieve lifelong wellness.** But I know that sometimes a book isn't enough.

Sometimes you need to talk with a real person who will help you cut through conflicting nutritional claims and keep your diet and exercise program on course. Someone who will remind you of your goals and help you celebrate your victories.

I'd like to be that person in your life. And to thank you for reading my book, I'm giving you the opportunity to **"test-drive" my health coaching service, risk-free.**

If you're ready to **take control of your health, call (858) 429-5750** in the San Diego area, or **(800) 557-0981** toll-free from anywhere in the United States, and mention the password **"EMPOWER."**

And if you have any questions, please don't hesitate to email **marilyn@lajollahealthcoach.com.**

In health,

Marilyn

Marilyn Beidler, C.N.C.
Founder of La Jolla Health Coach
Author of *Everyday Wellness: Fifty Simple Steps to Lifelong Health*

P.S. This offer may not be around forever. So if you're interested, **make the call right now before you forget!**

Are You Making These Nine Common Health Mistakes?

Download Your Free Report
from www.lajollahealthcoach.com/ew

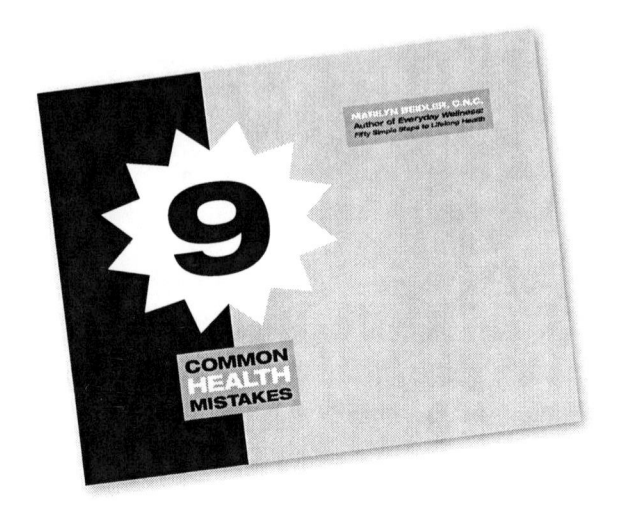